Intercultural Communication in Dentistry

Book **2** of the
Dental Communication
Brief Book Series

Toni S. Adams, RDH, MA

Odontocomm Productions

Rocklin, California

Artwork: Dreamstime.com

Published by:
Odontocomm Productions
Post Office Box 891, Rocklin, CA 95677

ISBN: 978-1-937535-01-8

Dedication

To the most important people
in my life:

John

You make everything possible.

&

Mom, Dad, Sean, Derek, Anya, & Katya

You inspire me to make you proud.

Acknowledgements

Thank you to the patients who I have been privileged to care for, and to the dental office colleagues who I was honored to work with. I have learned something valuable from every one of you.

Thank you to some extraordinary professors. You taught me about oral and written communication, culture, critical thinking, research, instruction, and training, and you inspired me to learn more and to share what I learned: Deanna Fassett, Rona Halualani, Mark Stoner, Marlene von Friederichs-Fitzwater, and Andy Wood.

Thank you to the Listers at Amysrdhlist.com for their daily posts that enlighten, inspire, enthuse, and amuse me every day.

Thank you especially to the many colleagues who have offered comments on various versions of these books.

Thank you, Tom Bentley, for your excellent editorial guidance (bentguy@charter.net).

Thank you, Cathy Seckman, RDH, for your countless valuable professional insights and indexing expertise (cathy@cathyseckman.com).

Introduction to the Dental Communication Brief Book Series

The topics in this series represent a fusion of the fields of dentistry and communication studies, especially health and intercultural communication.

After practicing for 26 years as a clinical dental hygienist, I returned to school to earn baccalaureate and master's degrees in Communication Studies. While at two universities as a senior senior and graduate student, I experienced many ah-ha! moments. I learned so much that I wish I had known while practicing.

The next best thing was to write The Dental Communication Brief Book Series so that others may benefit from my learning and new passion. The information in these volumes is meant for anyone who wishes to directly or indirectly improve communication in dentistry in order to enhance dental patient care. If you are a dental clinician, staff member, student, instructor, researcher, manager, trainer, company representative, or anyone interested in improving dental communication, then these books are for you.

Separate books allow readers to select the topics that interest them. These brief volumes can be read quickly, often in one or two sittings, so the information can be put to use immediately.

May your patients, your colleagues, and *you* benefit from your expanded communication knowledge.

Explore all the topics

Book 1. Health Communication/Persuasion in Dentistry
Communication skill is a key part of the dental armamentarium. Read about the elements and benefits of patient-centered care, the relationship between communication and evidence-based care, and both classic and new ideas about how to influence others.

Book 2. Intercultural Communication in Dentistry
Cultural issues complicate communication, especially as the United States and the world diversify. Learn about cultures, including your own, and how cultural matters influence dental interactions.

Book 3. Verbal Communication in Dentistry
Improve verbal competence and learn: how the words that we use impact practice; how to work with low literate (half of US residents) and limited English proficient (LEP) people and interpreters; about laws that mandate providing interpreters for LEP patients; and ideas for how to find and fund interpretation.

Book 4. Nonverbal Communication in Dentistry
As much as 92% of emotional communication, and a large proportion of other communication, is nonverbal. Emotions can run high in dentistry. What do we *say* to patients with our nonverbal messages, and what are they trying to *tell* us?

Book 5. Listening in Dentistry
The number one complaint of dental patients is that we don't listen to them. Learn why patients who feel heard are happier and healthier, and how to be a better listener.

Book 6. Patient Interviewing in Dentistry
This book addresses the purposes of health interviews and the skills needed to conduct them successfully, what patients want, cultural issues in interviewing, how to interview difficult people, and it also reviews motivational interviewing

Book 7. Patient Education in Dentistry
Learn about theories of learning, motivation, and decision-making; cultural issues; patient education strategies; teaching patients to search the internet; and how to minimize miscommunication.

Table of Contents

Learning Outcomes for Book 2   14

Introduction   17

Diversity and Health Disparities in the USA   19

Laws About Cultural Competence in Health   22

My Personal Experience With Culture   24

What Is Culture?   25

Culture as an Iceberg   26

Characteristics of Culture   28

     Culture is learned   28

     Culture is subtle and deeply ingrained   28

     Culture is dynamic   29

     Culture is variable   31

Acculturation and Culture Shock   32

Cultural Self-Awareness and the United States Culture   34

American Cultural Values   35

Cultural Principles   36

     Ethnocentrism   38

     Individualism and Collectivism   41

Individualism   41

Collectivism   42

Individualism meets collectivism   42

Times are changing   43

Context/Direct and Indirect Communication   44

Direct communication   45

Indirect communication   45

Direct communication meets indirect
communication   47

Chronemics and Cultural Time   49

Linear time   50

Holistic time   51

Linear time meets holistic time   51

How Do We Know About a Person's Culture?   54

Bringing It All Together   55

Rao and Physicians from Collectivistic
Cultures   55

Rao's conclusions   56

Saying the "C" word   57

Payer's Description of Healthcare in
Individualistic Cultures   58

The United States   60

France   61

Germany   63

Great Britain   64

Katalanos' Study of Southeast Asian Refugees   66

Seeking healthcare   67

Paying for healthcare   67

What is a prescription?   68

Views of disease and the body   68

Names   69

Cambodians   70

Hmong   70

Vietnamese   71

Conclusion   73

Glossary   75

Resources   79

References   81

Index   89

About the Author

Order Forms

Learning Outcomes for Book 2

- Understand the relationship between communication and culture in dentistry
- Appreciate culture's influence in health settings
- Begin cultural self-awareness exploration
- Be familiar with four cultural concepts
- Apply cultural concepts to various cultures
- Enhance intercultural communication skill

Intercultural Communication in Dentistry

Culturally effective health care is vital
and a critical social value.

-Committee on Pediatric Workforce, 2004

This isn't just politically correct,
it's good medicine.

-Voelker, *Journal of the American
Medical Association*, 1995

Humankind has not woven the web of life.
We are but one thread within it.
Whatever we do in the web, we do to ourselves.

-Chief Seattle

Introduction

A group of students and professors from the University of Wisconsin at Eau Claire School of Nursing presented a series of health education courses to Hmong (pronounced "Mong") immigrants. During the dental health unit, one immigrant described his culture's belief about how dental caries occur. "A very small bug with a big red head gets into the tooth and can only be killed by pulling the tooth out and crushing it and throwing it in the fire."[1] One nursing professor commented, "I felt humbled by the recognition of the narrowness of my knowledge of different cultures."

Many other cultural dental beliefs, customs, treatments, and folklore certainly exist, and many dental professionals are beginning to learn about them. Dental caregivers struggle with the challenge of communicating with and caring for people of all races, ethnicities, and cultural and personal backgrounds, just as all health care providers do, so there is always more to know about *culture* and its impact on the delivery of dental care. As you read this book and complete the activities you will enhance your understanding of **diversity** and expand your **intercultural communication competence**. However, I have two cautions.

First, do not assume that culture explains all behaviors. It is a huge part of life and explains a lot, but not everything. If someone is rude, insensitive, overbearing, or just plain nasty, perhaps it is because of his personality, or because he is unwell or fearful, or for other reasons, and not necessarily due to his cultural learning.

Second, do not expect to become experts by reading these few pages. The pursuit of intercultural

---

[1] Moch, Long, Jones, Shadick, & Solheim, 1999, p. 240

communication competence is a lifelong journey, not a single destination. No one can ever know everything about even a single culture, let alone all cultures or all people in them. We still try, however, because we have learned that the combination of study and experience bring us closer to the goal of understanding each other. To that end, this book outlines and illustrates four basic cultural concepts after first explaining in a little more detail how we, and our patients, can benefit when we know more about them.

Diversity and Health Disparities in the USA

We need only look around to realize that the world is changing. People travel more, move more, and immigrate more easily and more frequently than ever before. One in ten residents in the United States was born outside the country, and minority groups are the fastest-growing segments of the population. More than one in four residents are African-American, Hispanic, or Asian/non-Hispanic, a proportion that is estimated to increase to one in three by the year 2020, and to over one in two by 2050. "Minorities" became the "majority" in California in 1999. Almost 47 million Americans, 18%–or one in five of our population–speak a language other than English at home, and 21 million, or 8%, are limited in English proficiency. This diversification has expanded beyond the eastern, western, and southern edges of the country. It is becoming more prevalent throughout the nation, including the upper Midwest, New England, and the Rocky Mountain States.

Culture has a major influence on how healthcare is perceived and delivered, especially in this multicultural, multiethnic, multiracial, multireligious, multilingual tapestry of a nation, where minority groups suffer a disproportionate number of health problems compared to the majority. "All ethnic minority populations in the United States lag behind European Americans (whites) on almost every health indicator, including healthcare coverage, access to care, and life expectancy, while surpassing whites in almost all acute and chronic disease rates."[2]

Minority people also suffer excessively from dental diseases and the lack of resources to receive care. "Blacks,

---

[2] Kagawa-Singer & Kassim-Lakha, 2003, p. 577

Hispanics and American Indians/Alaska Natives have the poorest oral health of any population group in the United States."[3] Certainly many factors that contribute to these disparities are far beyond our control, but we can address them in part by enhancing our cultural knowledge and intercultural communication competence.

The extensive research on this topic has been reported in a wide variety of health literature and summarized in numerous government reports. Four reports are especially prominent and significant:

- The landmark Surgeon General's Report on *Oral Health in America* (2000) documented a "silent epidemic"[4] of oral diseases in the United States that impacts minority groups more than others.
- *Healthy People 2010*, the publication that enumerates the United States national health goals for the 2000–2010 decade, includes a chapter on health communication in which health professionals are urged to acquire the ability to "interact with diverse populations and patients who may have different cultural, linguistic, educational, and socioeconomic backgrounds."[5] (p. 11-11). *Healthy People 2020,* the health goal summary for the second decade of the 20th century, also focuses on culture in the *Health Communication and Information Technology* section. One objective relates to "providing new opportunities to connect with culturally diverse...populations."[6]

---

[3] Milgrom, Garcia, Ismail, Katz, & Weintraub, 2004, p 1391

[4] U. S. Department of Health and Human Services, 2000, p. 17

[5] U. S. Department of Health and Human Services, 2000, p. 11-11

[6] U. S. Department of Health and Human Services, 2010, retrieved January 20, 2011, from http://www.healthypeople.gov/2020/topicsobjectives2020/overview.aspx?topicid=18

- The Office of Minority Health issued *National Standards for Culturally and Linguistically Appropriate Services in Health Care* (2001), better known as the CLAS Standards. All entities, such as schools, hospitals, and clinics that receive government funding, must adhere to these standards, though all healthcare providers, including dental professionals, are also urged to follow them.
- The Health Resources and Services Administration produced an extensive report, *Transforming the Face of Health Professions Through Cultural and Linguistic Competence Education* (2005). This document looked at dentistry as well as medicine and concluded that healthcare disparities in the USA are not due entirely to access to care issues; patient and caregiver cultures and the culture of dentistry also play significant roles. As Cegala and Post pointed out, "Compared to Whites, minorities receive fewer tests, therapies, and procedures even after controlling for insurance status and access to regular primary care physicians."[7]

All of these reports mandate intercultural communication training for healthcare providers and their supporting staffs in order to prevent and treat disease, and to address disparities in the provision of health services.

---

[7] Cegala & Post, 2006, p. 854

Laws About Cultural Competence and Health

If national recommendations, standards, and policies, are not enough, some health providers are being legally compelled to learn about culture. As of this writing, California, New Jersey, and Washington have passed laws that obligate various healthcare providers to enhance their cultural knowledge and intercultural communication competence.

- California Assembly Bill 1195, that took effect on July 1, 2006, requires *all* continuing medical education, unless exempt,[8] to include cultural and linguistic competence materials in their curricula.
- New Jersey Senate Bill 144, 2004, requires cultural competence training as a condition of medical licensure.
- Washington Senate Bill 6194, 2005, requires *all health professionals* licensed in that state to take courses in multicultural health within basic education and continuing education.
- Arizona, Colorado, Florida, Georgia, Illinois, Kentucky, New Mexico, New York, and Ohio have introduced, discussed, and may be in the process of enacting their own versions of these laws. Georgia has considered requiring health providers to take a cultural competence course.

California, New Jersey, and Washington have not merely made recommendations or even issued policies; they have enacted *laws*. If this is happening in medicine, it is just a matter of time before it happens in dentistry. If it is

---

[8] Exemptions are granted only for courses that contain no clinical content, such as billing procedures

happening in a few states, it is just a matter of time before it extends to other states.

So, we have numerous ethical, professional, educational, personal, and, increasingly, legal reasons to learn about and understand diversity, culture, and intercultural communication, and to enhance our intercultural communication competence. These topics will be explored in this book, but they will also be integrated throughout all of the books in this series.

In this book, you will find a definition of culture and a discussion of its characteristics. You will begin your own cultural self-awareness journey, learn about four cultural principles, and see how those principles apply to specific cultures. Before proceeding, however, we will take a little detour. I believe that it is important for readers to understand that, even though I try to be objective, my prejudices may seep out, so at this point I want to share some of my own cultural story.

SIDEBAR: For more information on these laws and proposed laws see
- o culturalmeded.stanford.edu/news/laws.html
- o https://www.cme.ucsf.edu/AB1195.aspx
- o healthlaw.org
- o lep.gov

My Personal Experience With Culture

I am a 65-year-old white woman. I grew up in a military family, so during my childhood I lived all over the United States as well as in Germany and Turkey. As a young woman I was a flight attendant for an international airline and was fortunate to travel around the South Pacific and the Far East and work with people from all over the world. All in all, I have lived in 20 cities in 9 states and two other countries and traveled to many more cities, states, and countries. I spoke German as a child and have studied Latin and French. I practiced as a dental hygienist for 26 years in San Jose, California, during the time it was developing into one of the most diverse areas in the United States, so I worked with and cared for an array of individuals throughout my clinical career.

My purpose in sharing this information is not to toot my own horn. It is to make the point that, even though I had unusually extensive experience with many kinds of people in a variety of locations and contexts throughout my life, *I still did not understand diversity until I began to study it.* This is a critical point that I want to reiterate. Mere exposure to diverse individuals, while it may enhance sensitivity to difference, does not necessarily develop deep *understanding.* And, as it turns out, I am not alone. This is a common experience that is confirmed by intercultural communication research. Cultural principles cannot be understood through intuition; they must be studied and learned.

That study began for me when I retired from the clinical practice of dental hygiene and returned to school to earn bachelor and master's degrees in Communication Studies. Every course that I took included some cultural content, five courses addressed culture and intercultural communication exclusively, and I also read extensively outside of course requirements. I found these topics both fascinating and personally enriching, and finally realized how limited my own understanding had been. I encountered numerous "ah-ha" moments regarding past and current experiences, and in the process came to know myself better as well. I hope that this book helps you, the reader, to embark on a similar journey of discovery. I will begin with the basics.

What Is Culture?

What is culture? Definitions are plentiful. A Google search for "culture definition" produced over 3.8 million results! Edward T. Hall, considered the founding father of the study of intercultural communication, wrote simply, "Culture is communication" and "Communication is culture."[9] This elegant definition is more complex than it appears, so I developed an expanded definition.

Culture[10] is a subtle and constantly evolving pattern of learning that guides behavior, is passed from generation to generation, and includes social and religious structures, ways of communicating, thoughts, history, beliefs, values, roles, rules, and customs that are characteristic of groups of people.

This description defines culture broadly so that it is not necessarily limited to ethnic, racial, national, or religious groups. Any group that shares the components can be called a culture, and that includes dentistry.

---

[9] Hall, 1959, 1990, p. 94
[10] Words that are defined in the Glossary will appear in bold italics the first time they are discussed

Members of the dental field are both a subculture of medicine and host to numerous other subcultures of our own, which could include each specialty, each occupation, and even each individual office. Our field constantly evolves as new knowledge is incorporated into our training and practice, and that learning guides our behavior. Our history, language, beliefs, values, roles, rules, and customs are unique and set us apart from other groups. This analogy also applies to the various characteristics of culture, which I will explore after first describing a well-known cultural metaphor.

Culture as an Iceberg

Edward T. Hall was the first to write about what has become the most famous metaphor for culture—the iceberg. The obvious parts of culture, such as food and dress preferences, manners, customs, rituals, celebrations, taste, and even languages, are only the tip of the iceberg. The vast expanse of deeper and more meaningful cultural beliefs, values, attitudes, and assumptions that motivate the behaviors are mostly unseen and unknown, even to a group's own members.

We may notice that patients from some cultures will not make direct eye contact with us and then assume that this is a sign of deception or lack of connection, while for the patient it may be a sign of respect. A dental patient sees our lab jackets, masks, face shields, gloves, and other paraphernalia and may have a vague idea why we wear them, but is unlikely to have a deep understanding of infection control. A patient once told me that he thought the reason I used so many barriers and washed my hands so much was because I thought he was dirty. But infection-control practices are second nature to us and instantly understood by our dental colleagues. In both examples, observations of the tip of the iceberg combined with a lack of training resulted in misunderstandings.

Many articles and even courses that teach about culture focus mainly on surface characteristics. They may concentrate on lists of national and ethnic customs, rituals, foods, language, and other observable practices, but seldom touch on the immense, unseen, deep part of the iceberg. It *is* important, even critical, to know tip-of-the-iceberg information, especially for those who interact regularly with individuals from specific groups. However, I believe that a foundation of knowledge about a few general cultural characteristics and principles should be laid down first.

Therefore, in this book, I will begin with the **culture general** approach. That is, I will focus first on the foundations of culture, which will form a basis for the **culture specific** information about individual groups that follows. The culture general information will also assist you when you seek to expand your knowledge about other individual cultures on your own. Of course the two approaches often overlap and it is impossible to completely separate them, but, for the purposes of learning, that is what I will attempt to do here, beginning with culture's main characteristics.

Characteristics of Culture

Culture Is Learned

This is perhaps its most fundamental characteristic. Culture is not genetic or innate, but is passed from generation to generation. Newcomers gain knowledge from wiser and more experienced individuals as they grow up or grow into various cultures.

As we became acculturated into the dental field, we learned about its history, founders, the evolution of various techniques and philosophies, and even a new language. Ultimately, we graduated from our training programs and participated in a ceremonial rite of passage to indicate that we had learned and matured enough to be recognized as full-fledged members. Many of us, after we graduated and passed our board exams, were allowed to participate in another cultural ritual in which we changed our names: we added DDS, DMD, RDH, LDH, or RDA and began, literally, to expand our identities. The analogies are striking.

Culture Is Subtle and Deeply Ingrained

Erich Fromm, the well-known social psychologist, wrote, "Cultural factors influence the individual behind his back, without his knowledge."[11] Prominent intercultural researcher Geert Hofstede called culture, "the software of the mind."[12] As a white American, I believed that I did not

---

[11] Hall, 1959, 1990, cover
[12] Hofstede, 1997, title

have a culture. I thought that the idea of culture applied only to those who identified with particular ethnic, racial, religious, or national groups. I was wrong. *Everyone* has a culture. I just did not recognize my own culture precisely because it is so subtle and entrenched. Likewise, we who work in the dental field may not recognize that culture.

Dental colleagues have comparable values and follow similar practices that have become natural to us. We dress similarly for work, place greater value on oral health, and are often more fanatic about our personal oral care compared to the uninitiated. Our language includes formal terminology (microorganisms, microbes, bacteria, viruses), informal terminology (germs), and even slang (bugs). Sometimes we forget that not everyone understands our language or has the same values, so I think it is wise for us to occasionally step back and examine our dental culture.

Take time to think
How have your personal beliefs, values, attitudes, assumptions, and health practices changed as a result of your association with the dental field?

Culture Is Dynamic

Culture constantly evolves. The Greek philosopher Heraclitus (535–475 BCE) wrote "You can't step in the same river twice," and Thomas Wolfe (1900–1938) wrote a novel titled, *You Can't Go Home Again*. These authors, one ancient and one more contemporary, did not mean that the river or the home necessarily disappear, but rather that everyone and everything constantly change so the exact person can never again find the exact river or home.

Anyone who has ever moved from one place to another and then returned to visit "home" can confirm this notion. People change and come and go, structures are built and torn down, innovative technologies are introduced, new knowledge is applied, language evolves, and values are altered. Some may argue whether or not this constant evolution is "progress," but none can argue whether or not it occurs.

Dentistry has changed dramatically since I entered my first dental hygiene classroom in 1971. We follow a host of newer infection-control protocols, wear loupes and lights, make greater use of ultrasonic and piezo scalers, recommend powered toothbrushes and xylitol, take digital X-rays and intraoral photos, preserve enamel at all costs, use antimicrobials to treat periodontal disease, care for implants, use lasers and computers, and communicate with patients via email and social media. Every modern dental practice today has a website, which was unheard of in 1971.

Many of the changes are reflected in our language. We remove *biofilm* rather than *plaque*, we talk about *interdental care* rather than *flossing*, we attempt *remineralization* when possible rather than *restoration,* and we perform *debridement* rather than *root planing.* This list is long and I'm just getting warmed up, but you get the picture. I could never go back to my original dental "home." The school is still there, but it is not the same school, and I am not the same person.

Take time to talk
Ask someone who has been in the field longer than you to describe some of the changes she or he has experienced. Then discuss how those changes have contributed to the evolution of the dental culture.

Culture Is Variable

There is as much ***diversity*** within cultures as there is among them. *Diversity* refers to differences between and among members of a variety of cultures and can refer to sex, age, educational level and field, socioeconomic status, mental and physical ability, and many other variables in addition to race, ethnicity, culture, and language. Each person is unique, and they, like cultures, are complex, contradictory, and constantly evolving.

We all belong to numerous cultures that mesh with each other, or not. They combine and separate, intersect and interact to create distinct individuals. A person who belongs to a certain group can share race, ethnicity, national origin, geographic origin, history, *and* religion and yet still be different because of sex, age, personality, family, education, profession, and life experience. Just as individuals who were born and grew up in the United States vary greatly, so do those who travel and emigrate here.

People today are exposed to and influenced by numerous cultures. We enjoy food from all over the world, incorporate words from many languages, and adopt practices that originated in other countries. As an example, look at the broad interest in Asian philosophies and practices such as yoga and the martial arts. So we are all unique in our blend of personal characteristics, cultural assumptions, beliefs, values, attitudes, and practices.

Acculturation and Culture Shock

Acculturation, or the degree to which a newcomer assimilates and adapts to a new environment, is another important variable that relates to culture. It is difficult to be the new kid on the block, whether you move across town or around the world. We refer to the distress that people feel upon entering a new environment as **"culture shock,"**[13] a state of confusion, uncertainty, and anxiety that may cause us to long for familiar surroundings where things are done "right." Ultimately we adjust and adapt to the new place to some degree or other, and in the process may change our behavior and/or our attitudes and evolve into different individuals. Every person will change in a different way and thus acculturation is a major element that contributes to the variability within cultures.

We can experience a kind of culture shock when we change jobs or offices in the dental field. At first we are thrilled with the new environment and the positive differences compared to the previous position. Then we begin to have problems. We may find that our new coworkers use variations of the language and apply the art and science of patient care differently. The new office may be disorganized where we had been organized, or out of date where we had worked hard to stay current. We gradually adapt, perhaps finding that the new ways are preferable in some cases or changeable in others. In the process we learn and grow as professionals and as individuals. This same progression occurs more or less whenever people are faced with change.

So far we have found that culture is acquired through learning, and that it is subtle, deeply ingrained,

---

[13] Kluykanov, 2005

constantly changing, and filled with difference. Now you may be surprised to learn that the next step in increasing cultural knowledge involves looking inward.

Cultural Self-Awareness and the United States Culture

If we want to understand other cultures, we must first understand our own. "All that one ever gets from studying foreign culture is a token understanding. The ultimate reason for such study is to learn more about how one's own system works....an achievement of gargantuan proportions for anyone."[14] The effort is worth it. Sondra Thiederman, a cultural expert, states that such study enhances our pride, helps us recognize our own core values and assumptions, and so helps solidify our identities.

This important exploration results in two main outcomes. First, we begin to realize how profoundly cultural assumptions influence behavior, and second, we come to appreciate that others may have different assumptions, so we are less likely to judge their behavior based on our values. Since the full exploration of our own cultural identities is an enormous task, the purpose of this section is merely to introduce the topic.

Here I will discuss why we know so little about the American culture, briefly summarize some of what we do know, and refer you to two websites with exercises that can start you on your own pursuit of cultural self-awareness. I hope that this brief discussion offers insight to Americans as well as to those who are trying to understand us.

There are two main reasons why we don't know very much about our own culture. First, we tend to think of culture as something that belongs only to others and as a result may not think of it as worthy of our attention. As I stated earlier, for most of my life I did not think that I

---

[14] Hall, 1959, 1990, p. 30

personally had a culture or that we as Americans had a culture. I was wrong on both counts.

Second, it is only relatively recently that social scientists and the public press have begun to focus on the American culture, a "new" topic. "This neglect implies that Americans do not have rituals, magic, elaborate kinship systems, reciprocal gift-giving customs, child-rearing practices, curing rites, feuds, disputes, myths, legends, beliefs about ghosts, or any other behaviors and beliefs common to cultures in the rest of the world."[15] But of course our culture includes all of these elements and more. We may not view them as parts of culture just because practices seem less exotic when viewed from the inside compared to when they are viewed from the outside.

American Cultural Values

What are some American values? What traits do we admire and what personal characteristics do we value? Several authors who have tried to define the American culture have concluded that these traits and characteristics include: independence, individuality, freedom, self-reliance, equality, friendliness, hard work, education, generosity, wealth, privacy, cleanliness, efficiency, initiative, "can do" attitude, competition, and fair play, among many others.

Do we *all* value all of these traits to a similar degree? Of course we don't. This is the same in every culture and illustrates what I already discussed; there is as much diversity within a single culture as there is among different cultures. Are all of these values applied uniformly? Of

---

[15] Rynkiewich & Spradley, 1975, pp. 1–2

course they aren't. We say we value equality, but we know that all is not equal in the United States, and certainly not in the provision of healthcare.

Even though these general terms have their descriptive limitations, they do ring true most of the time to most Americans. Please note the presence of these characteristics and their counterparts in the discussion of cultural principles later in this book.

There is another path to cultural self-awareness. "One of the most effective ways to learn about oneself is by taking seriously the cultures of others. It forces you to pay attention to those details of life which differentiate them from you."[16] So the two processes complement each other. The study of personal cultures helps us understand others, and the study of other cultures helps us understand ourselves. Win-win.

---

[16] Hall, 1959, 1990, p. 31

Take time to read and think and talk
This three-part exercise may take some time, but the investment will be worth the effort.
1. Reread the list of American values from the previous paragraph. Do you agree with this list? What values would you add or remove? Discuss your choices with friends.
2. Visit the following websites and answer some of the questions regarding your personal culture. Compare notes with friends from the same and different cultures.
    a. Look at this excerpt from the book, *Developing Cross-Cultural Competence: A Guide to Working With Children and Their Families* edited by Eleanor Lynch and Marci Hanson (1998, 2nd ed.). Scroll to the bottom of the page, or read all of this insightful and informative writing: http://clas.uiuc.edu/fulltext/cl08481/cl08481.html#3
    b. Look at Sondra Thiederman's perceptive article on why and how to become more culturally self-aware: http://www.thiederman.com/articles_detail.php?id=37
3. Read more about the American culture. Find ideas at toniadams.com–>Resources & Links–>American Culture.

Cultural Principles

Now that we have begun to increase our personal cultural awareness, we are ready to study some basic ideas about culture. Scholars from all over the world have developed dozens of cultural principles, theories, models, and concepts. I have chosen to write about the four of these that I believe are most related to dental care: *ethnocentrism*; *individualism and collectivism*; *context* or *direct* and *indirect communication*; and *time*.

Ethnocentrism

Ethnocentrism, the idea that one person's beliefs, values, attitudes, and practices are superior and preferable to those of any other person or group, is probably the only trait that is common among most cultures. The idea is also timeless. At around 400 BCE, Aeschylus wrote, "Everyone's quick to blame the alien."[17]

William Sumner, an American anthropologist, appears to have coined the term and published the first formal definition in 1906:

> Ethnocentrism is the technical name for this view of things in which one's own group is the center of everything, and all others are scaled and rated with reference to it....Each group nourishes its own pride and vanity, boasts itself superior, exalts its own divinities, and looks with contempt on outsiders. Each group thinks its own folkways the only right

---

[17] Knowles, 1999, p. 6

ones, and if it observes that other groups have other folkways, these excite its scorn.[18]

Sumner argued that ethnocentric beliefs are central to the survival of a culture and to understanding difference among cultures. After all, if we did not think that our beliefs, values, and practices were right, true, and good, then we would change them and they would eventually evolve in some way or die out completely.

Sumner listed numerous examples. Many cultures refer to their members as "human beings" or "the people," implying that others are not human. The early Chinese called themselves "The Middle Kingdom," because those in the center are the most important. Ancient Greeks, Romans, and Middle Easterners referred to all outsiders as "barbarians," and Jewish people have traditionally referred to themselves as "the chosen people." The early natives in Greenland thought that Europeans were sent to them to learn proper manners. "Each state regards itself as the leader of civilization, the best, the freest, and the wisest, and all others as inferior." [19] As a result, most cultural groups believe that the reason for their existence is to civilize the rest of humanity.

Ethnocentrism is also personal. My grandmother used to say, only half-jokingly, "Everyone's crazy but me and thee—and sometimes I'm not too sure about thee." In other words, if you don't believe and do as I believe and do then you are crazy. How ethnocentric!

We can imagine the difficulties that may result in healthcare when both patient and caregiver feel that their views are right and true and the other's opinions are wrong and false. Steven Dowd and his colleagues, authors of a culture textbook for nurses, were more blunt, "Health care

---

[18] Sumner, 1906, p. 13
[19] Sumner, 1906, p. 14

professionals must recognize that their way may not necessarily be the best for the client and should not disregard other people's ideas as 'ignorant.'"[20]

We who have been trained in Western healthcare systems tend to value science over intuition, whereas in many other cultures it is the opposite, and those two orientations can collide. Therefore, it is important to understand the concept of ethnocentrism, and especially to recognize it in ourselves, in order to deliver patient-centered care. When we do not understand this concept we limit our ability to build relationships with patients, comprehend and appreciate their views, and find common ground.

Other cultural concepts expand on the notion of ethnocentrism and describe some of the specific differences that, as Sumner wrote, "excite our scorn." The following three cultural theories are not hard and fast. They are, as one favorite professor used to say, "theories, not laws." They vary within cultures and within individuals, so please remember that my descriptions focus on the far ends of each spectrum for the purposes of learning. I caution against assuming that any individual falls neatly into any category. That would be stereotyping. Additionally, in this time of globalization, it is impossible to know how life experiences have influenced the values and preferences of any person. The purpose of studying these distinctions is to increase awareness of their existence so we can begin to understand a variety of views.

---

[20] Dowd, Giger, & Davidhizar, 1998, p. 119

Individualism and Collectivism

Geert Hofstede, a Dutch social scientist and pioneer intercultural communication researcher, developed the cultural dimensions of **individualism** and **collectivism**. These concepts together are described as: the degree to which the preferences, interests, customs, rules, and goals of the group take precedence over those of the individual. Collectivism predominates in Asia, Africa, the Middle East, southern Europe, Latin and South America, as well as in island and native cultures, whereas individualism is seen mostly in North America and northern Europe.

Individualism

Individualistic cultures focus on "I." They value independence, uniqueness, and competition, so that the needs and preferences of each person usually come before those of the group. Self-sufficiency is an asset and dependence on others is not respected. Association with a particular group is not central to a person's identity, success, or survival, and, even more, individualists are *expected* to have strong personal identities. Since equality is valued, people feel that everyone should be treated alike.

The United States has been called the most individualistic culture in the world, but most minority groups within the US tend to be more collectivistic. We are a nation of mostly immigrants and their offspring, so we tend to reflect the orientations of our forefathers, which may fall anywhere on the individualism-collectivism spectrum.

Collectivism

Collectivistic cultures focus on "we." Groups in these cultures are strong and cohesive and offer security and acceptance in exchange for absolute loyalty from members. The needs and interests of the group are central to life and always take priority over those of any single member, so the focus is more on *inter*dependence, harmony, conformity, and collaboration. Group affiliations are essential to the identity, success, and even the survival of its members. Without the group, the individual is insignificant. Outsiders are judged against the beliefs, practices, and values of the group and strangers are not trusted until they can prove themselves worthy, which may take years.

Collectivist in-groups can differ from culture to culture. In Africa the group is the community, in Japan it is the company, and in Latin and Asian cultures it is the family. The term "family" can include both nuclear and extended families and may even incorporate ancestors in some Asian families and honorary family members such as godparents in Latin families. A Mexican-American friend told me that she could not understand why many American families move and separate so easily, even to accept a better job or to upgrade a home. She would not consider living away from her extended family for any reason.

Individualism meets collectivism

Collectivist cultures tend to be hierarchical, so preference is given to members of the in-group, especially those of higher rank who are usually older males. The concept of "first come, first served," common among individualists, translates in collectivist cultures to the higher status or in-group person comes first. In the dental office this could mean that a traditional high status person from a collectivist culture might expect preferential treatment.

Individualists value personal opinions and feel comfortable voicing them. Collectivists strongly prefer consensus and so state the group's feelings only after agreement is reached. That is why collectivists may not make immediate decisions about dental treatment but wait instead until they can consult with other group members, especially those in the upper levels of their hierarchies.

The notion of pride is also seen differently. Individualists generally appreciate personal acknowledgement and awards. Collectivists, on the other hand, may be uncomfortable with individual praise, which they feel should reflect upon and honor only their groups. A friend who immigrated from an Asian country told me that it would make her uncomfortable to hear someone tell her that she has pretty eyes, but she would be very happy to hear that all the women in her family have pretty eyes. In the dental office a collectivist child who has done well with his home care might be embarrassed to hear, "You can be proud of yourself," but might respond more positively to, "Your family can be proud of you."

Times are changing

Globalization and international business experience have changed the corporate culture and conflict-resolution styles in different parts of Asia. Twenty years ago in China and Taiwan the style was more yielding and compromising, traditional in collectivist cultures. But now the style can be much more confrontational, as it is in individualistic societies. Young people in Japan, rather than conforming to group norms as their collectivist parents expect, are increasingly asserting their individuality in such ways as wearing Mohawk hairstyles or dyeing their hair different colors so that older people have taken to calling them *"foreigners."*[21]

Vandello and Cohen studied collectivism in the United States, where individualism predominates. They concluded that Alaska, Hawaii, California, and the southern states from coast to coast show a much stronger tendency toward collectivism compared to the rest of the country. On the other hand, Davis and Konishi studied whistle-blowing among Japanese nurses. We might think that strong collectivist loyalties in Japan would prevent such behavior because it could interfere with group harmony. However, the practice has increased to the extent that laws have been enacted to protect whistle-blowers.

Remember, the distinctions between individualism and collectivism are not absolute; they represent a range of orientations that are present in all cultures to varying degrees. The purpose of learning about them is not to label people, but rather to draw attention to possible differences. This is only the beginning of many ways that people can be different.

Context/Direct and Indirect Communication

Culture has a profound influence on the way we communicate. Edward T. Hall defined the extremes of that difference as **high context** and **low context**. He described **context** as the degree to which the setting influences the message. This idea involves more than just the physical surroundings, but also includes the people who are involved, their relationships with the environment and each other, the time and timing of a given interaction, and other

---

[21] J. Hwang lecture, October 26, 2005

factors. Storti renamed these dimensions **direct** and **indirect communication** respectively, which are the terms I will use here.

Direct and indirect communication, like individualism and collectivism, are opposite ends of a spectrum with countless variations in between. Direct communication generally predominates in individualistic cultures, and indirect communication is usually linked with collectivism, so each is associated with the same areas of the world noted in the previous section.

Direct communication

People in North American and northern European cultures tend to communicate directly. That is, we tend to be precise and give a lot of verbal detail in a conversation. We prefer to "tell it like it is" and "give the facts, Ma'am, just the facts." Most of our meaning is in the words that we speak, so it is important to express disagreement, say what we mean, and mean what we say. Direct communication is even more pronounced in scientific fields such as medicine and dentistry. We cannot imply scientific facts; we must state information as specifically, clearly, and completely as possible.

Indirect communication

Where indirect communication predominates, on the other hand, much of the meaning in a conversation is implied rather than stated explicitly, and participants must fill in the blanks. This implicit meaning is transmitted mainly through different types of nonverbal communication, including physical appearance, movement, touch, vocal expression, and the use of time, space, and distance.[22] The ultimate goal in an encounter is not only to exchange information, but mainly to maintain harmony (a collectivistic characteristic), so people avoid confrontation and may or may not say what they mean or mean what they say.

A perfect example of indirect communication is the Korean concept of *nunch'i*, which literally means, "eye measured."[23] Nunch'i refers to the ability to instinctively size up a situation or a person. Beyond "reading" actions and grasping messages, it also includes a deep understanding of a person's underlying motivations and emotions. *Nunch'i* must be mutual; the first person must send an understandable message and the second person must correctly interpret it.

Take time to try it
Those who favor direct communication also use indirect communication, and sarcasm is a good example. Say, "I hate you" as if you mean it and then sarcastically as a joke. Same words, opposite meanings, all implied through vocal inflection and timing.

---

[22] For more information, see Book 4 in the Brief Book Series, *Nonverbal Communication in Dentistry.*
[23] Robinson, 2003, p. 57

Direct communication meets indirect communication

In cultures that rely heavily on indirect messages, certain words may mean the opposite of their dictionary definitions. "No" is only implied, and "yes" can mean "no." When I visited Japan and asked a taxi driver to take me to a certain attraction that he knew had been closed, he replied, "Ahhhh, this is difficult." If I had understood the Japanese culture and the concept of indirect communication, I would have realized that this meant, "no."

According to several friends who speak Chinese, there is no single, direct way to say "no" in the Chinese languages, though there are numerous indirect ways. On the other hand, "yes" may mean "I hear you but I don't agree," or "I do not understand but I don't want to embarrass myself by saying so," and not necessarily, "I understand" or "I will do as you ask."

Cambodian people tend to answer "no" to a negative question because to them it confirms the statement. Katalanos reported an actual conversation. The Cambodian participant was interviewed afterward to determine his meaning (which is written in parentheses):

Healthcare provider: You didn't take your pills.

Cambodian patient: No. (That is not right, I did take them.)

Healthcare provider: Don't you want to get well?

Cambodian patient: No. (That is not right, I do want to get well).[24]

Imagine the confusion that this type of interaction might cause in the dental office.

---

[24] Katalanos, 1994, p. 37

An indirect communicator may appear to agree to follow through with home care instructions when that was not what he meant at all. A dentist from a high context culture was having trouble with several staff members who dressed too informally for his taste. The office manager spoke with them but nothing changed, so she suggested that the dentist himself should speak with them. The dentist's reply when confronted with this plan reveals a person who relies on indirect communication. He said, "they should just know." That statement expresses the essence of indirect communication.

Of course we can have indirect communication relationships in a direct communication culture and vice versa. My husband and I have been married for 42 years and can convey a wealth of information with a mere look or raised eyebrow. Some long-time dental colleagues may also be on the same wavelength. On the other hand, even in places where indirect or implied communication is more common, some information must be precise, such as in business or science.

So, as with individualism and collectivism, the concept of directness of communication is not exact. We can find other examples of direct and indirect communication in the way that we use a precious commodity, our time.

Chronemics and Cultural Time[25]

The way we use time is a form of nonverbal communication and its study is called **chronemics**. Time is probably *the* most precious commodity in the practice of healthcare. The amount of time needed to wait for the caregiver or patient, to conduct an interview, to deliver or receive treatment, for treatment to take effect, to get a prescription, to see a specialist, to feel better, and to heal are all of intense interest to patients and practitioners. The way we use time is often a function of our cultures. Edward T. Hall, an anthropologist who lived and worked in many different parts of the world, developed the concepts of monochronic and polychronic time.

 Monochronic time orientation, found generally in individualistic cultures such as those in northern Europe and North America, is a more linear view that focuses on accomplishing tasks one at a time. **Polychronic time orientation**, more commonly seen in collectivistic Asian, Latin, island, native, American Indian, African, Mediterranean, and Middle Eastern cultures, tends toward a more circular or holistic perspective and focuses on personal relationships. For simplicity, I will refer to monochronic time as **linear time**, and to polychronic time as **holistic time**.

---

[25] A version of this section also appears in Book 4, *Nonverbal Communication in Dentistry*, because the subject of Cultural Time is fundamental to both books.

Linear time

From a linear perspective, time is thought of as a commodity, an actual thing that we can give, take, invest, budget, spend, spare, save, waste, use, lose, or lend. The same verbs could be applied to money. In North American dental offices, time *is* money, time flies, and we always seem to be in a time crunch. We have specific rules about being on time, who can be kept waiting, and for how long. The rules differ for higher status people. It is all right for the boss or the professor to be late for work or class, but not all right for the employee or the student.

"Business before pleasure," as we often say in the United States, means that task and social needs should be separate and that the task is more important. Business meetings are conducted point-by-point according to agendas, and dental clinicians see patients one at a time. If a person has a dental appointment at 1:00, regardless of her status, she is expected to show up by 1:00. We hate interruptions because they interfere with our agendas. We focus on privacy and individuality and are more concerned with being "on" time.

The ever-present clock represents a linear time culture. The clock seems to rule our lives. It dictates when we rise in the morning, when we go to sleep at night, and most of what we do in between. We are even a bit disoriented when we cannot find a clock, such as in theaters, malls, and restaurants.

I recently noticed that we have sixteen clocks in our house, six in our kitchen alone. We didn't actually go out and buy all of those clocks as such, though we did buy a few. The reason that we have so many clocks is because almost every appliance and gadget that we purchase comes equipped with one.

The clock also rules our business lives. Appointment times must be honored almost to the second or at least the rule, "first come, first served," must be followed. And as we are served we expect to have the exclusive attention of the clerk or businessperson. But not everyone thinks of time this way.

Holistic time

People with a holistic time orientation tend to think of time as more fluid and almost limitless. Task and social needs are combined and several events can occur simultaneously. Schedules are flexible and there is no such thing as an interruption because relationships with people come before agendas. Holistic-timers are ruled by an internal clock and are more concerned with being "in"[26] time.

In holistic time cultures business is conducted very differently compared to the rigid schedules in linear cultures. An appointment at 1:00 doesn't necessarily mean 1:00. A holistic time person just "knows" (*indirect communication*) that a 1:00 appointment really means 1:30 or 2:00, or even later, and does not expect undivided attention from a proprietor. The businessperson greets and speaks with several people at a time, deals with both personal and business issues at once, and seems in no hurry to conclude any deals. There is very little privacy in this scenario. Since multiple matters are attended to at the same time in the presence of all, everyone's business often becomes everyone's business.

Linear time meets holistic time

Linear time and holistic time orientations are not always distinct or exclusive to certain cultures or countries. Even in the predominately linear time-oriented United

---

[26] Storti, 1999

States, we tend toward linear time in business and holistic time in the home and in social situations, and women and men tend more toward holistic and linear time orientations respectively. Japan is an exception among Asian cultures and can be even more linear time-oriented than we are in the United States, with events so tightly scheduled that there is hardly a moment to take a breath. In spite of these exceptions, most people usually identify more strongly with one orientation or the other, the difference is usually one of degrees, and the important thing is to recognize that there is a difference.

Not surprisingly, both linear and holistic time people are frustrated when they try to function in the other person's culture. My husband and I became friends with a couple who had recently moved from Hong Kong and we were invited to their home for dinner. We arrived at the appointed time, 6 PM sharp, with flowers and a box of candy for our hosts. The couple was startled, even astonished, to see us. The husband was vacuuming the living room, the wife was wearing curlers and a robe, and dinner had not been started. There was plenty of embarrassment to go around.

Janet MacLennan, a Canadian, wrote about her experience living and teaching at a university in Puerto Rico, including her adjustment to a holistic time culture. She felt that she was making progress when she purposely arrived one hour "late" for her dog's appointment with the veterinarian. No one at the vet's office even noticed.

In North American dental offices we earn our livings with appointments as we try to adhere to demanding schedules. Everyone expects promptness. Patients can become annoyed, offended, or even angry when they are kept waiting past their scheduled appointment times. We practitioners can be frustrated as we try to stay on time and also fulfill our ethical and legal responsibilities to provide excellent care. People who arrive late make it difficult to do that.

I cared for four sisters who had emigrated from the Philippines. These charming women also became personal friends, but, from my linear time perspective, they were eternally late for their dental appointments. They would joke with me that they were on "Filipino time." I did not always appreciate the humor, especially when I was delayed in seeing my other patients. (A Hawaiian friend says that they refer to a holistic time orientation as, "Island Time.")

I don't know the solution to the conflict between linear time and holistic time orientations in the dental office. However, I did find that as my friends became more acculturated to life in the United States, they began to understand my predicament and started to arrive more promptly, though the process took years. I have begun to lose some of my concern over the issue since studying and beginning to understand the differences between linear and holistic time orientations.

How Do We Know
About a Person's Culture?

The last three cultural concepts that I discussed are related to each other. Individualism, direct communication, and linear time orientation are usually found in the same cultural groups, as are collectivism, indirect communication, and holistic time orientation.

The next logical question is, "How do you determine a person's time orientation?" The answer is, of course, that you cannot, just as it is impossible to determine precisely where a person may fall on the ethnocentrism, individualism-collectivism, or directness of communication continua. We cannot expect to know what even an individual may not know, especially due to the inconsistent, complex, and constantly evolving nature of culture. To complicate the issue even more, these categories and definitions represent only a few of the cultural principles that scholars have described. There are many more ways to be different, but even these four can combine and interact to create a wide variety of possible orientations in any single person.

The important thing to remember is that, just as heredity or diet or homecare may or may not influence certain dental conditions, these concepts may or may not influence behavior and the decision-making processes in the dental office. They are, however, significant factors to consider, and, when understood, can offer insights for patient care.

Bringing It All Together

In order to demonstrate the principles at work, I will now switch to a culture specific approach and overview three sources that compared and contrasted individual cultures: Nagesh Rao's survey of physicians in three collectivistic cultures; Lynn Payer's comparisons of healthcare in four individualistic cultures; and Nikki Katalanos' study of the health beliefs and practices of recent refugees[27] from Southeast Asia.

Rao and Physicians from Collectivistic Cultures

During his five-year study, Nagesh Rao interviewed 91 physicians in three different countries. In his essay, *"Half-truths" in Argentina, Brazil, and India: An Intercultural Analysis of Physician-Patient Communication,"* he tried to answer the question, "How do physicians in different countries communicate with culturally diverse patients?"[28] He developed three main conclusions and one argument.

---

[27] Please note the difference between refugees and immigrants. Refugees move from one country to another, usually involuntarily, because of dramatic events that endanger their lives. Immigrants typically move from one country to another by choice and design, which may nevertheless be a difficult and extensive process.

[28] Rao, 2003, p. 313

Rao's conclusions

Rao argued that an interaction between a physician and a patient is always intercultural, even when both people are of the same ethnic and national culture. Other researchers came to the same conclusion. They even called the medical culture a barrier to physician-patient communication, especially in intercultural settings, due to differences in educational levels, language including medical jargon, values, socioeconomic status, gender, race, religion, and time orientation. Of course this can also be an issue in dentistry. The effort to set aside our ethnocentrism and personal and professional cultures when treating people with different beliefs is surely a challenge.

All four of the cultural principles that I discussed are represented in Rao's three conclusions. First, he noted that all of the physicians described their countries as diverse. One Brazilian doctor expressed it well, "You have many countries inside a country."[29] The presence of *ethnocentrism*, a nearly universal trait that is magnified in the midst of diversity, is implied in this statement. In his second conclusion, Rao noted that the physicians treated the family as the patient because they felt that personal and family identities were inseparable, which reflects the interdependence of *collectivism*.

Third, Rao reported that 90% of the physicians stated that if a patient's life were threatened by an illness or injury, they would not immediately tell the patient. They reasoned that to do so would harm the patient psychologically and so reduce the person's ability to cope with the condition. The doctors preferred instead to inform family members first so that they could support the patient and/or reveal the information gradually over a span of

---

[29] Rao, 2003, p. 313

several visits. Rao called this strategy "half-truths,"[30] another way to say *indirect communication*. The fact that there seems to be no hurry to reveal the diagnosis reflects a *holistic time orientation*.

Saying the "C" word

Other research confirms Rao's third conclusion. Holland, Geary, Marchini, and Tross surveyed physicians from 20 countries and areas of the world. Oncologists from Africa, France, Hungary, Italy, Japan, Panama, Portugal, and Spain reported that they preferred not to say the word *cancer* when making a diagnosis. They substituted it with words like *swelling* or *inflammation*, which is another example of *indirect communication*.

This practice brings up all sorts of ethical, legal, and practical issues for healthcare providers in the United States, where we have laws about patient privacy and informed consent. When we treat patients from cultures where this practice is common, we need to remember at least two things. First, they may not know all of their medical histories, especially if they are new to our country. Also, their families may expect to be completely informed about their conditions, perhaps even before the patients are.

In Book 3 of the Brief Book Series, *Verbal Communication in Dentistry*, I tell the story about a Russian man who had terminal cancer, but had not been told about his diagnosis. An interpreter, in the course of doing his job, revealed the man's condition to him. The man's son was furious. "Do you understand what this means to a Russian man? It means you've just given him a death sentence. He is going to lose all hope, he's going to stop eating, he's going to

---

[30] Rao, 2003, p. 314

stop drinking, he's just going to curl up in a corner and die. You've just ruined two years of us carefully hiding this from him."[31]

What is the answer to this sticky situation for American healthcare providers? We are torn between our legal and ethical obligations on one side, and differing cultural views on the other. I'm not sure that there is a universal answer, but at least now we know that this difference can exist. Now I turn to the opposite ends of the cultural spectra to look at reports on healthcare and beliefs in countries that tend toward individualism, direct communication, and linear time orientation.

Payer's Descriptions of Healthcare in Individualistic Cultures

Lynn Payer was an American biologist, physiologist, and medical journalist based in Europe. She spent ten years studying cultural influences in healthcare in four First-World countries and documented her findings and conclusions in her book, *Medicine and Culture*. She chose to focus on England, France, West Germany[32], and the United States because of their similar life expectancy and infant mortality rates and because she could speak all of the languages. Her research, though she admitted that it was based mostly on personal accounts, was still extensive and used all the documentation that she could find in addition to numerous interviews.

---

[31] Dohan & Levintova, 2007

[32] Payer's original research in 1988 looked at West Germany when it was a separate country from East Germany. She followed up in 1996, after the two had been reunited. For brevity, I will refer to both as "Germany."

The British medical community had great respect for Payer and her research, which was evident in her prominent obituary in the *British Medical Journal*. She "challenged the popular view that medicine was grounded in objective science....(and) showed how cultural values and opinion profoundly influenced medical practices."[33]

Payer's investigation began when she was diagnosed with a grapefruit-sized uterine fibroid tumor while in France. Her French physicians recommended a myomectomy (removal of the tumor only, a procedure that could take up to six surgeries but would preserve her uterus), whereas her American physicians automatically recommended a complete hysterectomy. This striking difference of medical opinions piqued her interest so she began her research. Payer ultimately found that French doctors performed about one-third the number of hysterectomies per capita compared to American doctors.

According to what we have learned so far, England, France, Germany, and the United States all tend toward individualism, direct communication, and a linear time orientation, but Payer found many shades of difference within those categories. While she admitted that there were many similarities among the countries, she contended that the differences were more interesting and revealing. She discovered that, among many other variations, the exact same symptoms might be diagnosed differently depending on the country in which they were found.

I will focus on three main areas of difference discussed in the book: each country's general philosophy toward healthcare, represented by its most valued action; main focus of health concern; and **wastebasket diagnoses**. Payer coined the term *wastebasket diagnosis* and defined it as a catch-all cause or condition that people think explains most of their vague and relatively mild symptoms, such as

---

[33] Newman, 2001, p. 871

aches and fatigue, that cannot be attributed to any other cause.

Payer's book was originally published in 1988 with an update in 1996. I will discuss the 1988 findings for each country and then note changes that may have been reported in the newer edition. Please remember that there is as much difference within cultures as there is among them and that the generalizations summarized here are far from absolute.

The United States

According to Payer, probably the best single modifier to describe American healthcare is *aggressive*. We Americans want to *do*, we focus on germs, and we usually blame unexplained symptoms on viruses. Doing something is always better than doing nothing and most of us do not value physicians or patients who want to wait and see. We commonly say, "There must be something that we can *do*," and "What are we waiting for, let's *do* something." My father used to say, "*Do* something, even if it's wrong!" We prefer surgery to medication, but if we use medication we tend to use high doses of the strongest drugs.

Americans use two metaphors that relate to the notion of aggressiveness in healthcare. First, illness is war. War requires strong measures that are reflected in our language. Illness is the "enemy" that we want to "fight" and "conquer," we look down on people who don't "battle" the "opponent," and in order to do so we use an "armamentarium." "The patient who 'beats' cancer is considered superior to the patient who fights but succumbs, who is in turn superior to the patient who refuses to fight."[34]

---

[34] Payer, 1988, pp. 132–133

Second, the body is a machine. A machine must be maintained with regular check-ups and the components can be fixed or replaced. We have developed the ability to transplant and implant many body parts including artificial teeth. The heart is the ultimate machine and in the United States coronary bypass surgery is performed up to 28 times as often as it is in some parts of Europe.

Americans focus on germs and our *wastebasket diagnosis* is *a virus*. When we have the sniffles or just don't feel well we say, "I just have a little virus," which usually means, "I have something but I don't know exactly what it is." Since we always want to *do* something and *fight* the illness, we think that when we cannot "beat" the "invaders" that we have "failed." When a patient doesn't show up for an appointment, we call that a "failure." A cancer patient who does not improve after chemotherapy is said to have "failed." An American physician is likely to think of a patient's death as a "failure."[35] And we dental caregivers tend to think that if our patients don't improve then either they or we have "failed." Since we are as ethnocentric as the rest of the world, this approach to healthcare seems natural to us. However, it is not the same in Europe.

France

Where Americans are aggressive and favor *doing*, the French favor *thinking*. They minimize reliance on evidence-based findings and instead favor reflection and theorizing, which is a legacy of their Cartesian heritage. René Descartes was the famous French philosopher who said, "Cogito ergo sum," (I think therefore I am), which placed "intellectual elegance"[36] above systematic research in the French medical psyche. Cartesianism in French medicine was

---

[35] Rao, 2003
[36] Payer, 1988, p. 40

explained to Payer as, "If the idea is good, the body has to follow."[37]

A new, supposedly revolutionary flu vaccine had been introduced while Payer was researching in France, but was criticized by American doctors because randomized controlled trials had not been done. Jacques Monod, then head of the Pasteur Institute that had developed the drug, told Payer, "I am very confident about vaccinating large numbers of people without challenge experiments."[38] Remember that, in spite of this opinion, the infant mortality and life expectancy rates were about equal in all four of the countries that Payer studied.

According to Payer, the French *wastebasket diagnosis* has to do with liver problems. The national illness before the 1980s was *crise de foie* (liver crisis) and, though this emphasis has softened, the liver and bile duct are still considered the sources of many health problems. "Fragile liver" and "fragile bile duct" are still common diagnoses, and many drugs including aspirin and antibiotics are dispensed as suppositories so the medications will not pass through the liver.

The French also place great emphasis on the **terrain**. This difficult-to-translate term relates to a person's constitution and the body's natural ability to fend off disease, but it is more than what we refer to as the immune system. In France, a great deal of effort is placed on bolstering the terrain by taking tonics and vitamins and by making sure that the body is rested.

French doctors tend to be more conservative in all of their treatments compared to American doctors, preferring instead "medicines douces" (gentle therapies).[39] A "French

---

[37] Payer, 1988, p. 40
[38] Payer, 1988, p. 39
[39] Payer, 1988, p. 65

dose" of medicine is about half that of an "American dose,"[40] but doctors are still likely to recommend homeopathy, aromatherapy, or a stay at a spa before prescribing antibiotics. The French and American cultural approaches to medicine also contrast with the German and British approaches.

Germany

German medicine, according to Payer, has been strongly influenced by Romanticism, a philosophical, musical, and artistic movement from the 1800s that emphasized feeling over thinking. So, the Americans *do*, the French *think*, and the Germans *feel*. Payer was told that Germans, contrary to the stereotype, are emotional and romantic but just don't show it. This view includes a belief in the healing powers of nature, and so Payer found that the use of spas, homeopathy, and herbalism are even more common than in France and also include other "natural" treatments such as long walks in the forest and mud baths.

Germans are especially concerned with the heart and blood pressure. Their wastebasket diagnosis is **herzinsuffizienz**[41], a mild heart insufficiency that, in its more advanced stages, might be called heart failure, but really has no exact translation into other languages. A companion problem to herzinsuffizienz is low blood pressure. During the time Payer was conducting her research, the German formulary listed 85 drugs to treat *low* blood pressure. The same blood pressure readings that would make most Americans physicians happy are considered pathological and treated with medications in Germany.

---

40 Payer, 1988, p. 66
41 I don't even try to pronounce this word!

The Germans combine the use of the "natural" treatments mentioned above with the use of an extraordinary number of prescription drugs. Payer reported that at the time of her research the German formulary included 120,000 medications compared to 1,180 in Iceland. No statistics for other countries were given, but this meant that Icelanders had access to less than 1% the number of medications compared to Germans.

German doctors also commonly prescribe medications in combination; it is not unusual for a patient to be taking 15 drugs to treat one condition. Patients have more opportunity to receive prescriptions because they visit their doctors more than twice as often (about 12 times per year) compared to patients in Britain (5.4 times per year), France (5.2 times per year), and the United States (4.8 times per year). Of those drugs, digitalis (as of 1988) was one of the most prescribed; it was used not only to treat heart disease, but also "as a general tonic"[42] to prevent it. The view of health in Great Britain represents a fourth perspective.

Great Britain

Payer's research on Great Britain revealed yet another unique national health character. The British tend to take a *wait and see* attitude in regards to health, focus on their bowels, and concern themselves with constipation and **autointoxication**. They approach healthcare with the same reserved stereotype for which they are famous, and "do less of nearly everything,"[43] including fewer screening exams, tests, X-rays, and surgeries. Because they do less screening, fewer people are considered sick. They prescribe fewer drugs and in lower doses compared to Americans,

---

[42] Payer, 1988, p. 84
[43] Payer, 1988, p. 101

including recommending lower doses of vitamins. Payer found that the philosophy of the National Health Service *reflected* a British tendency to be conservative, to keep a stiff upper lip, and to feel that the good of the society should come before individual needs, not the other way around.

British people tend to be stoic and expect self-control of themselves and others. Even though medication use overall in Britain is lower, tranquilizers are actually prescribed more compared to the other countries. They are dispensed for the most part to help "overactive" people, but are even prescribed for depression. Many of those "overactive" people actually want tranquilizers to help them fit in with an ascetic and self-reserved society. An offshoot of the self-control issue has led to exceptional skill in the fields of anesthesiology and control of pain. British anesthesiologists are internationally respected and looked to as leaders in the field.

Another issue related to self-control is concern about the bowels. Payer quoted an editorial from the *British Medical Journal*, "From infancy, the British are brought up to regard a daily bowel action as almost a religious necessity,"[44] and people take pride in such control. The British wastebasket diagnosis is *constipation*, defined as anything less than a daily emptying of the bowels. It is believed that constipation brings on a condition called *autointoxication*, or absorption into the body of "toxins" from the bowels. Payer told the story of a British prep school where every morning the boys were required to answer the matron's question, "Been?"[45] Those who were honest or stupid enough to answer "no" were treated to a laxative.

---

[44] Payer, 1988, p. 116
[45] Payer, 1988, p. 118

Payer found many fundamental differences among the four groups that she studied. Without her insights, we might have gone on thinking that healthcare in these countries that are usually lumped together and called individualistic was mostly similar. Now we see that the Americans want to *do* and focus on viruses and germs; the French prefer to *think* and are most concerned about the liver and the terrain; the Germans *feel* and tend to blame many ills on heart, blood pressure and circulation issues along with Herzinsuffizienz; and the British like to *wait and see* and are fastidious about bowel actions, constipation, and autointoxication.

Payer's newer edition reported relatively few changes to her original conclusions. Americans were beginning to turn to alternative types of medicines more frequently and women with breast cancer were more likely to be offered relatively conservative treatments. But overall the Americans were still aggressive and the British still conservative and the main concerns in the four countries remained virtually the same. Now, for further contrast, I turn to a study of people from the opposite side of the world.

Katalanos' Study of Southeast Asian Refugees

Katalanos studied the health beliefs and practices of Southeast Asians who settled in New Mexico, and reported her findings in her master's thesis titled, *When "Yes" Means "No."* She focused on the Vietnamese, Cambodian, and Laotian/Hmong groups. Most were newly arrived refugees who had lived through horrors to get to the United States, so they were relatively unacculturated and still reeling from their experiences. Some of the people that she studied may have been here longer and had a greater chance to adjust to the United States, or they may have been the children of the original refugees, so, once again, don't assume that everyone from these countries shares the same characteristics that Katalanos describes. I summarize her study here to illustrate the similarities and differences among groups of people that we usually lump together as collectivists, "Asians," and "Southeast Asians."

Seeking healthcare

Almost all of the refugees that Katalanos studied shared the experience of losing their homes and many family members before coming to the United States, and they all had difficulty adjusting to our way of delivering healthcare. Because of financial limitations, lack of transportation, inability to take time off work, and other barriers, and because of their cultural history of not having had access to healthcare, many Southeast Asians sought out health professionals only as a last resort. As a result, they were usually sicker when they finally saw physicians.

Paying for healthcare

The way that Americans pay for healthcare was also different and difficult for these refugees. Many lacked money or insurance and were used to bartering or giving food as a gift in return for services. They may have thought that the food gift they brought to the caregiver was payment for the service, whereas the caregiver may have thought of it as a nice gift but then sent them to collections for nonpayment. A subsequent notice from a collection agency may have caused such deep shame that they never returned.

Dealing with prescriptions

Another issue had to do with medications. The idea of a prescription was unknown. When the refugees did go to a doctor who recommended a medication, they were used to receiving it on the spot and not having to go to another place and pay extra for it. They may also have been disappointed when no medication was dispensed at an appointment, regardless of the diagnosis or lack of one.

They tended to think of American medications as too strong for them, so they may have taken less than the prescribed dose and, as a result, either did not improve or were prescribed a larger dose or a stronger medication. A lot of them preferred home remedies to medical remedies. Many home treatments were ancient and either worked well or were harmless and may have helped the people feel better emotionally and psychologically.

Views of disease and the body

They looked at disease differently. Ideas about the causes of disease came from a combination of Animism, Buddhism, and ancient Chinese medicine. Physical illness resulted from accidents (causing such problems as broken bones, cuts, food poisoning) and infections (resulting in malaria, tuberculosis, cholera, and so forth). Metaphysical illnesses, related to the principles of Yin and Yang, were caused by bad wind, hot and cold energy imbalances, poor diet, and excessive emotion. Supernatural illnesses resulted from soul loss or the influence of bad spirits. Soul loss in particular was believed to be a major cause of supernatural illness within the Hmong community.

Compared to Westerners, they viewed certain parts of the body, including the eyes, the blood, and the head differently. They believed that direct eye contact was a sign of aggression, or at least rudeness, and Cambodians especially thought that it caused illness. To the Southeast Asians, blood represented energy, and some believed that it could not be replenished, so they wanted to avoid any kind of blood loss at all.

Katalanos learned that the head was a source of life for all of the groups, and that it was extremely personal and mostly untouchable. The Lao/Hmong in particular believed that to touch the head caused soul loss and the Vietnamese believed that only an elderly person could touch a child's head. A casual acquaintance, even a healthcare provider who has extra latitude, should not ruffle a child's hair or pat her on the head.

Take time to think and talk
What implications do these beliefs about the body have in the dental office? Ask friends for their ideas and compare and contrast yours with theirs.

Names

The groups also differed in regards to naming. For all groups, the family name came first, before the given name, which represented the importance of the family over the individual (collectivism), but each culture differed in other ways. Cambodians historically had only one name, but were forced to take second names by the French. For the Vietnamese, the middle name may have indicated the person's sex. For the Hmong, women may or may not have taken their husbands' names when they were married, and titles were used with given names. So Diana Jones would have been called, "Dr. Diana" or "Mrs. Diana" rather than "Dr. Jones" or "Mrs. Jones." This was a sign of respect because personal names had deep meaning. But these naming customs were not universal among the Hmong because different tribes may have done things differently, another example of the heterogeneity within groups. To complicate things even more, some individuals may have changed the order of their names as an adaptation to life in the United States, so it is understandable that Americans can get confused about Asian names. If you are uncertain, ask the person.

Cambodians

The Cambodians suffered perhaps the most devastating traumas of the three groups, so were more likely to be depressed, which they may have denied because to them it was a shameful condition. Overall, they tended to be formal but friendly, "slow moving, patient, and easy-going."[46]

They were the most class-conscious of the three groups, having immigrated from a country that had historically had four classes: royalty, upper class, middle class, and lower class, each with a different language. So when trying to find an interpreter for traditional Cambodians, it was necessary to find someone from the same class. They honored the right hand but did not value the left hand, so found it rude to hand something to another person with the left hand. They tended to answer *no* to a negative question. To them, it confirmed a statement.[47]

Hmong

The Lao, mostly Hmong, had the strongest belief in American medicine of the three groups. The major difference when comparing them to Cambodians and Vietnamese was that there was less male domination among the Hmong and so they valued having a girl child

---

[46] Katalanos, p. 36
[47] Refer to the conversation transcribed in the discussion of indirect communication earlier in this book

more than the others. Women were respected as the moral and ethical experts and family treasurers.

They believed that each person had 36 souls. The most inferior soul lived in the feet, the next most important was just above, moving up the body so that the most important soul resided in the head. One of the rudest things a person could do was to touch another person with an inferior part of her or his own body. So they would not touch another person's shoulder with a hand, and would never put a hand on someone else's head. Fortunately for dental caregivers, they made an exception for healthcare providers. They also felt that pointing a finger was rude, but that pointing or even showing the bottom of a person's foot was the highest insult.

Vietnamese

Of the three groups, the Vietnamese were the most likely to use Chinese healthcare practices and folk medicines. They believed that people should soften their voices; a loud voice was considered disrespectful and even aggressive and would leave a lasting impression.

The Vietnamese had strict customs regarding intersexual touching. A man could not offer to shake a woman's hand, and could only shake hands if she offered first. Strangers and slight acquaintances, even healthcare providers, should not put their arms around a person's shoulders (such as when leading a person to an operatory) because this was considered disrespectful, especially if a man touched a woman in this way. Husbands would not even touch their wives in public, yet it was commonplace for same sex friends to hug and hold hands, and this did not imply homosexuality as it did in the United States.

Among the Vietnamese, direct communication was considered rude, embarrassing, and disrespectful; they preferred indirect communication. Katalanos suggested using "a soft voice and....innuendos."[48] On the other hand, it was not considered rude to ask a person's age or salary or the price of an item that someone had purchased. These questions represented interest in and respect for the person and helped the asker to gauge the other person's character. However, the direct question could be answered indirectly.

Smiles had many meanings: happiness/sadness, understanding/misunderstanding, agreement/disagreement, sickness, fear, "stoic self protection,"[49] or all of these at once. They considered it a sign of respect to dress up for a doctor's appointment, and a healthcare provider who dressed too casually may have been thought to show disrespect to the patient.

All in all, Katalanos found numerous similarities and differences among the Southeast Asian refugees that she worked with and studied, and her insights add to our understanding of all the cultural concepts discussed in this book.

_____

[48] Katalanos, 1994, p. 29
[49] Katalanos, 1994, p. 32

Conclusion

We have looked at a wide variety of people and cultures. Rao studied physicians from mostly collectivist cultures; Payer studied patients and physicians in mostly individualist cultures; and Katalanos looked at traditional Southeast Asian refugees who had recently immigrated from, and were still very close to, their collectivist roots.

The findings and conclusions from these three researchers provide excellent illustrations of the differences both within and among groups. I have included only brief summaries of their findings and strongly urge readers to explore more about individual cultures of interest, including and perhaps beginning with, your own. As Hammerschlag, a physician and psychiatrist who cared for and lived among American Indians for most of his career, wrote,

> What we see as science, the Indians see as magic. What we see as magic, they see as science. I don't find this a hopeless contradiction. If we can appreciate each other's views, we can see the whole picture more clearly.[50]

I conclude this book with a quote from Irene Gonzales, RN, PhD, CNP, a nursing professor at San Jose State University. She wrote a letter from the viewpoint of a minority patient from a collectivist culture who had been severely injured in a car accident and had just been released from the hospital after five weeks. Though this letter does not refer to a dental patient, there are many parallels that apply to our care. Dr. Gonzales' last two paragraphs are especially poignant.

---

[50] Hammerschlag, 1988, p. 14

Thank you for treating me and my family as a unique and vital part of the healthcare team. Even though I may appear very different from you on the outside or may respond to situations in a different way, I am still very much the same on the inside. You have demonstrated your care for me by how you treated my family and me during this very stressful time.

Yes, even though I can't speak or understand English, I can definitely tell you how very grateful I am—with every fiber of my being—that you have given a piece of your life to me. Maybe someday you will need my help and I can be there for you. Stop and listen carefully. What you hear is our hearts and spirits connecting forever.

Respectfully and gratefully,
Your Patient for Today[51]

That sums up what we are all about when we care for all kinds of people. Culture frames our lives and gives us rules to live by. We are mistaken when we assume that everyone has the same rules and then judge others based on that assumption. Culture is an integral part of, and profoundly influences, how illness is experienced and how we practice as healthcare providers. We cannot check our cultural learning at the door when we enter a dental office. Our cultures are with us always, even at work, so it is critical to understand our own and other cultures as well as possible.

---

[51] Gonzales, 2002, p. 49

Glossary

Acculturation: The degree to which a newcomer assimilates and adapts to a new environment

Autointoxication: According to Payer, to a British person, a condition brought on by constipation in which toxins from the bowel are absorbed into the body

Chronemics: The study of time in relation to culture. (Also see *linear, holistic, monochronic,* and *polychronic time orientations*)

Collectivism: Refers to cultures in which the needs and interests of the group take priority over those of the individual people. (Also see *Individualism*)

Context: The degree to which the setting, participants, time, timing, and other factors influence communication. (Also see *high context, low context, direct communication,* and *indirect communication*)

Cultural general approach to study: A broad approach to studying culture with a focus on understanding general characteristics and principles

Cultural specific approach to study: A focus on studying individual cultures separately.

Culture: A subtle and constantly evolving pattern of learning that guides behavior, is passed from generation to generation, and includes social and religious structures, ways of communicating, thoughts, history, beliefs, values, roles, rules, and customs that are characteristic of groups of people

Culture Shock: The distress that people feel upon entering a new environment

Direct communication: Interaction in which much of the message is verbally precise and detailed because less information is implied by the surroundings. Edward T. Hall originally referred to it as *low context*. (Also see *context* and *indirect communication*)

Diversity: Refers to differences between and among members of a variety of cultures and can refer to sex, age, educational level, profession, socioeconomic status, mental and physical ability, and many other variables in addition to race, ethnicity, culture, and language

Ethnocentrism: The concept that a person's own beliefs, values, attitudes, and practices are superior and preferable to those of any other person or group

Herzinsuffizienz: According to Payer, to a German person, this is a mild heart insufficiency that in its more advanced stages might also be called heart failure

High context: Edward T. Hall's original term for *indirect communication.*

Holistic time orientation: A circular view of time that focuses on relationships and is more commonly seen in collectivistic cultures. Edward T. Hall originally referred to it as, "polychronic time." (See also: *monochronic* and *linear time orientations)*

Immigrant: Person who moves from one country to another by choice and design (Compare to *Refugee*)

Indirect communication: Interactions in which much of the message is implied by the participants, their relationships, the setting, and other nonverbal features. Edward T. Hall originally referred to it as *high context*. (Also see *context* and *direct communication*)

Individualism: Refers to cultures in which the needs and interests of individual people take priority over those of the group as a whole. (See *Collectivism*)

Intercultural Communication Competence: The ability to set aside one's ethnocentrism, communicate with honor and respect, and attempt to understand others in spite of diversity

Linear time orientation: A direct view of time that focuses on accomplishing tasks and is more commonly found in individualistic cultures. Edward T. Hall originally referred to it as, "monochronic time." (See also *polychronic* and *holistic time orientations*)

Low context: Edward T. Hall's original term for *direct communication*

Monochronic time orientation: Edward T. Hall's original term for *linear time orientation*

Polychronic time orientation: Edward T. Hall's original term for *holistic time orientation*

Refugee: Person who moves from one country to another, usually involuntarily, because of dramatic life events that endanger her/his life. (Compare to *Immigrant*)

Terrain: According to Payer, to a French person this means constitution, or the body's natural ability to fend off disease

Wastebasket Diagnosis: According to Payer, a catch-all cause or condition that people think explains most of their vague and relatively mild health symptoms, such as aches and fatigue, that cannot be attributed to any other cause

Resources

Readers can find lists of resources and many links to more information online. I did not include them in this book because they can become obsolete so quickly. Additionally, it is much easier to click on the link and go directly to the source rather than trying to retype the URL.
Go to toniadams.com–>Resources & Links.

These categories of information are on the website:
- American Culture
- Children and Teens
- Cultural Self-Awareness
- Culture
- Culture and Health
- Dental and Medical Dictionaries, Encyclopedias, Glossaries
- Dental and Medical Topics Assortment
- Diabetes
- Forms
- Government, Foundation, and Other Organization Reports
- Health Law Regarding Language
- Health Literacy
- Medications
- Multiple Language Materials
- Plain Language and Caring for Limited English Proficient Patients
- Research, Data, Statistics
- Special Patients
- Translation Aids
- Translation and Interpretation Issues

References

Airhihenbuwa, C. O., & Obregon, R. (2000). A critical assessment of theories/models used in health communication for HIV/AIDS. *Journal of Health Communication, 5*(Suppl.), 5–15.

Beamon, C., Devisetty, V., Forcina Hill, J. M., Huang, W., & Shumate, J. A. (2005). A guide to incorporating cultural competency into medical education and training. *National Health Law Program*. Retrieved July 11, 2008, from http://www.healthlaw.org/library

Beebe, S. A, & Biggers, T. (1986). The status of the introductory intercultural communication course. *Communication Education, 35*, 56–60.

Brislin, R. (1993). *Understanding culture's influence on behavior.* Fort Worth: Harcourt Brace College Publishers.

Burgoon, J. K., Buller, D. B., & Woodall, W. G. (1996). *Nonverbal communication: The unspoken dialogue* (2nd ed.). New York: The McGraw-Hill Companies, Inc.

Cegala, D. J., & Post, D. M. (2006). On addressing racial and ethnic health disparities: The potential role of patient communication skill interventions. *American Behavioral Scientist, 49*, 853-867.

Committee on Pediatric Workforce (2004). Ensuring culturally effective pediatric care: Implications for education and health policy. *Pediatrics, 114*, 1677–1685.

Connolly, I. M., Darby, M. L., Tolle-Watts, L., & Thomson-Lakey, E. (2000). The cultural adaptability of health sciences faculty. *Journal of Dental Hygiene, 74*, 102–109.

Datesman, M K., Crandall, J., & Kearney, E. N. (1997). *The American Ways: An introduction to American culture* (2nd ed.). White Plains, NY: Longman.

Davis, A. J. & Konishi, E. (2007). Whistleblowing in Japan. *Nursing Ethics, 14*, 194–202.

Dhir, I., Tishk, M. N., Tira, D. E., & Holt, L. A. (2002). Ethnic and racial minority students in U.S. entry-level dental hygiene programs: A national survey. *The Journal of Dental Hygiene, 76*, 193–201.

Dohan, D., & Levintova, M. (2007). Barriers beyond words: Cancer, culture, and translation in a community of Russian speakers. *Journal of General Internal Medicine, 22*(Supp.2), 300–305.

Dowd, S. B., Giger, J. N., & Davidhizar, R. (1998). Use of Giger and Davidhizar's transcultural assessment model by health professions. *International Nursing Review, 45*, 119–122, 128.

Fitch, P. (2004). Cultural competence and dental hygiene care delivery: Integrating cultural care into the dental hygiene process of care. *The Journal of Dental Hygiene, 78*, 11–21.

Garcia, R. I. (2005). Addressing oral health disparities in diverse populations. *Journal of the American Dental Association, 136*, 1210, 1212.

Gibson, S., & Zhong, M. (2005). Intercultural communication competence in the healthcare Context. *International Journal of Intercultural Relations, 29*, 621-634.

Gonzales, I. (2002). Even though I don't speak English: A letter to every healthcare provider. *Critical Care Nurse, 22*(4), 47–49.

Gudykunst, W. B., & Lee, C. M. (2002). Cross-cultural communication theories. In: W. B. Gudykunst and B. Mody (Eds.), *International and intercultural communication* (2nd ed., pp. 25–50). Thousand Oaks, CA: Sage Publications.

Hall, E. T. (1959, 1990). *The silent language.* New York: Anchor Books.

Hall, E. T. (1983; 1989). *The dance of life.* New York: Anchor Books.

Hall, E. T. (2000). Context and meaning. In L. A. Samovar & R. E. Porter (Eds.), *Intercultural communication: A reader* (9th ed., pp. 34–43). Belmont, CA: Wadsworth Publishing Company.

Hall, E. T., & Hall, M. R. (2002). Key concepts: Underlying structures of culture. In J. N. Martin, T. K. Nakayama, & L. A. Flores (Eds.), *Readings in intercultural communication experiences and contexts* (2nd ed., pp. 165–172). Boston: McGraw Hill.

Hammerschlag, C. A. (1988). *The dancing healers: A doctor's journey of healing with Native Americans.* San Francisco: Harper.

Hofstede, G. (1997). *Cultures and organizations: The software of the mind.* New York: McGraw-Hill.

Holland, J. C., Geary, N., Marchini, A., & Tross, S. (1987). An international survey of physician attitudes and practice in regard to revealing the diagnosis of cancer. *Cancer Investigation, 5*, 151–154.

Huff, R. M., & Kline, M. V. (1999). Health promotion in the context of culture. In D. J. Huff & M. V. Kline (Eds.), *Promoting health in multicultural populations: A handbook for practitioners* (pp. 3–22). Thousand Oaks, CA: Sage Publications.

Katalanos, N. L. (1994). *When yes means no: Verbal and nonverbal communication of Southeast Asian refugees in the New Mexico health care system.* Unpublished masters thesis, University of New Mexico, Albuquerque.

Klyukanov, I. E. (2005). *Principles of intercultural communication.* Boston: Pearson Education, Inc.

Kagawa-Singer, M., & Kassim-Lakha, S. (2003). A strategy to reduce cross-cultural miscommunication and increase the likelihood of improving health outcomes. *Academic Medicine, 78*, 577–587.

Knowles, E. (Ed.). (1999). *The Oxford dictionary of quotations* (5th ed.). Oxford: University Press.

Kreps, G. L., & Thornton, B. C. (1992). *Health communication theory & practice* (2nd ed.). Prospect Heights, IL: Waveland Press, Inc.

Leeds-Hurwitz, W. (1990). Notes in the history of intercultural communication: The Foreign Service Institute and the mandate for intercultural training. *Quarterly Journal of Speech, 76*, 262–281.

Lyman, R. (2006, August 15). New data shows immigrants' growth and reach. *The New York Times*, A–1.

Luckman, J. & Nobles, S. T. (2000). *Transcultural communication in health care.* Albany, NY: Delmar.

Ludenia, K., & Donham, G. W. (1983). Dental outpatients: Health locus of control correlates. *Journal of Clinical Psychology, 39*, 854–858.

MacLennan, J. (2002). There's a lizard in my living room and a pigeon in my classroom: A personal reflection on what it takes to teach in a different culture. *Journal of Intercultural Communication Research, 32*, 13–28.

Magee, K. W., Darby, M. L., Connolly, I. M., & Thomson, E. (2004). Cultural adaptability of dental hygiene students in the United States: A pilot study. *The Journal of Dental Hygiene, 78*, 22–29.

Milgrom, P., Garcia, R. I., Ismail, A., Katz, R. V., & Weintraub, J. A. (2004). Improving America's access to care: The National Institute of Dental and Craniofacial Research addresses oral health disparities. *Journal of the American Dental Association, 135*, 1389–1396.

Moch, S. D., Long, G. L., Jones, J. W., Shadick, K., & Solheim, K. (1999). Faculty and student cross-cultural learning through teaching health promotion in the community. *Journal of Nursing Education, 38*, 238–240.

Morey, D. P., & Leung, J. J. (1993). The multicultural knowledge of registered dental hygienists: A pilot study. *Journal of Dental Hygiene, 67*, 180–185.

Network Omni: Multilingual Communications (2006). *Caring with CLAS: Cultural competence in health care.* Author. Retrieved October 13, 2007, from http://www.dhh.louisiana.gov/offices/miscdocs/docs-90/Caring%20with%20CLAS%20-%20Legislative%20Fact%20Sheet.pdf

Newman, L. (2001). Lynn Payer. *British Medical Journal, 323* (7317), 871.

Northouse, L. L., & Northouse, P. G. (1998). *Health communication: Strategies for health professionals.* Stamford, CT: Appleton & Lange.

Payer, L. (1988, 1996). *Medicine and culture: Varieties of treatment in the United States, England, West Germany, and France.* New York: Henry Holt and Company.

Rao, N. (2003). "Half-truths" in Argentina, Brazil, and India: An intercultural analysis of physician-patient communication. In L. A. Samovar, & R. E. Porter (Eds.), *Intercultural communication: A reader* (10th ed., pp. 309–319). Belmont, CA: Wadsworth.

Regis, D., Macgregor, I. D. M., & Balding, J. W. (1994). Differential prediction of dental health behaviour by self-esteem and health locus of control in young adolescents. *Journal of Clinical Periodontology, 21*, 7–12.

Rhine, R. D. (1989). William Graham Sumner's concept of ethnocentrism: Some implications for intercultural communication. *World Communication, 18*, 1–10.

Robinson, J. H. (2003). Communication in Korea: Playing things by eye. In L. A. Samovar and R. E. Porter (Eds.), *Intercultural communication: A reader* (10th ed., pp. 57–64). Belmont, CA: Wadsworth/Thomson Learning.

Rogers, E. M., Hart, W. B., & Miike, Y. (2002). Edward T. Hall and the history of intercultural communication: The United States and Japan. *Keio Communication Review, 24*, 3–26. Retrieved May 8, 2006, from http://www.mediacom.keio.ac.ip/publication/pdf2002/review24/2/pdf

Roter, D. L., & Hall, J. A. (1993). *Doctors talking with patients/patients talking with doctors: Improving communication in medical visits.* Westport, CT: Auburn House.

Rynkiewich, M. A., & Spradley, J. P. (1975). The Nacirema: A neglected culture. In: M. A. Rynkiewich & J. P. Spradley (Eds.), *The Nacirema* (pp. 1–5). Boston: Little, Brown and Company.

Sartory, G., Heinen, R., Pundt, I., & Johren, P. (2006). Predictors of behavioral avoidance in dental phobia: The role of gender, dysfunctional cognitions and the need for control. *Anxiety, Stress and Coping, 19*, 279–291.

Shin, H. B., & Bruno, R. (2003). Language use and English-speaking ability: 2000, Census 2000 brief. *U.S. Census Bureau, U.S. Department of Commerce, Economics and Statistics Administration.* Retrieved August 12, 2008, from http://www.census.gov/prod/2003pubs/c2kbr-29.pdf

Sisty-LePeau, N. (1993). Oral healthcare and cultural barriers. *Journal of Dental Hygiene, 67*, p. 156.

Smedley, B. D., Stith, A. Y., & Nelson, A. R., 2003 (Eds.). Executive summary of *Unequal treatment: What healthcare providers need to know about racial and ethnic disparities in healthcare.* Washington, DC: The National Academies Press. Retrieved October 23, 2005, from http://www.nap.edu/catalog/10260.html

Storti, C. (1999). *Figuring foreigners out: A practical guide.* Boston: Intercultural Press.

Sumner, W. G. (1906). *Folkways.* Boston: Ginn and Company.

Thiederman, S. (2005). *American culture: Knowing yourself in order to understand others.* Retrieved November 7, 2005, from http://www.thiederman.com/articles_detail.php?id=37

Triandis, H. C. (2003). Culture and conflict. In L. A. Samovar, & R. E. Porter (Eds.), *Intercultural communication: A reader* (10th ed., pp. 18–28). Belmont, CA: Wadsworth.

U.S. Department of Health and Human Services (2000). *Healthy people 2010: Understanding and improving health* (2nd ed.). Washington, DC: U.S. Government Printing Office.

U.S. Department of Health and Human Services, National Institute of Dental and Craniofacial Research, National Institutes of Health (2000). *Oral health in America: A report of the Surgeon General: Executive summary.* Rockville, MD: Author. Retrieved June 17, 2005, from http://www.nidcr.nih.gov/AboutNIDCR/SurgeonGeneral/

U.S. Department of Health and Human Services, Health Resources and Services Administration (2005). *Transforming the Face of Health Professions Through Cultural and Linguistic Competence Education: The Role of the HRSA Centers of Excellence.* Rockville, MD: Author. Retrieved May 14, 2007 from http://www.hrsa.gov/culturalcompetence/curriculumguide/default.htm

U.S. Department of Health and Human Services, Office of Minority Health (2001). *National standards for culturally and linguistically appropriate services in health care: Executive summary.* Rockville, MD: Author. Retrieved October 23, 2005, from www.omhrc.gov/assets/pdf/checked/executive.pdf

Vandello, J. A. & Cohen, D. (1999). Patterns of individualism and collectivism across the United States. *Journal of Personality and Social Psychology, 77,* 279–292.

Voelker, R. (1995). Speaking the languages of medicine and culture. *Journal of the American Medical Association, 273,* 1639–1641.

Wanning, E. (2000). *Culture Shock! USA.* Portland, Oregon: Graphic Arts Center Publishing Company.

Yamaguchi, Y., & Wiseman, R. L. (2003). Locus of control, self-construals, intercultural communication effectiveness, and the psychological health of international students in the United States. *Journal of Intercultural Communication Research, 32,* 227–245.

Index

A

Acculturation, 32–33, 75
Aeschylus, 38
American culture, 33–37
Autointoxication, 64, 65, 75

C

Cambodians, 68–69, 70
Cancer, using word for, 57–58
Cegala, D., 21
Chronemics, 49, 75
CLAS standards *(National Standards for Culturally and Linguistically Appropriate Services in Health Care)*, 21
Collectivism, 42–44, 55–58, 75
Communication
  competence in intercultural, 17–18
  direct, 45, 47–48, 76
  indirect, 45–48, 57, 76
  nonverbal, 45–46
  verbal, 45–48
Context, high and low, 44, 75, 76, 77
Cultural competence, 22–23
Culture
  American, 33–37
  context in, 44–45
  defined, 25–26, 75
  and dental beliefs, 17
  determining, 54
  diversity in, 31
  dynamism of, 29–30
  effects of globalization on, 43–44
  ethnocentrism in, 38–40
  general, 27, 75
  iceberg as metaphor for, 26–27
  individualism, collectivism in, 41–44
  influence on healthcare, 19, 74
  learned, 28
  personal story of, 24

specific, 27, 75
subtlety of, 28–29
Culture shock, 32–33, 75

D

Davis, A., 44
Dentistry, as a culture, 17, 28, 30
Descartes, René, 62
Direct communication, 45, 47–48, 76
Diversity
    within cultures, 31
    defined, 76
    and health disparity, 19–21
    in physician study, 56
    understanding, 24–25
Dowd, Steven, 38

E

Ethnocentrism, 38–40, 56, 76
Eye contact, 68–69

F

France, healthcare in, 61–63, 66
Fromm, Erich, 28

G

Germany, healthcare in, 63–64, 66
Globalization, affecting culture, 43–44
Gonzales, Irene, 73–74
Great Britain, healthcare in, 64–66

H

"Half-truths in Argentina, Brazil, and India: An Intercultural Analysis of Physician-Patient Communication, 55
Hall, Edward T., 25, 26, 44, 49, 76
Hammerschlag, C., 73
Head, as source of life, 69
Health disparities, in U.S., 19–21
Healthcare
    comparison study of, 58–61
    culture's influence on, 74

in France, 61–63, 66
in Germany, 63–64, 66
in Great Britain, 64–66
paying for, 67
in Southeast Asia, 66–72
in the United States, 60–61, 66
Healthy People initiatives, 20
Heraclitus, 29
Herzinsuffizienz, 63, 76
Hmong people, 17, 69, 70–71
Hofstede, Geert, 28, 41
Holistic time, 51–53, 57, 76

I

Iceberg, as culture metaphor, 26–27
Immigrant, 55n27, 76
Indirect communication, 45–48, 57, 76
Individualism, 41, 42–44, 76
Intercultural communication, 17–18
Intercultural competence, in communication, 20–21, 77

K

Katalanos, N., 47, 66–69, 71–72, 73

L

Lao/Hmong people, 69, 70–71
Laws, on cultural competency, 22–23
Linear time, 50–53, 77

M

MacLennan, Janet, 52
Medications, prescriptions
    Americans using, 60
    Britons using, 64–65
    the French using, 62
    Germans using, 63–64
    Southeast Asians using, 68
Medicine and Culture, 58
Minorities, oral health of, 19–20
Monochronic (linear) time orientation, 48, 77
Monod, Jacques, 62

N

Naming, 69–70
National Standards for Culturally and Linguistically Appropriate Services in Health Care (CLAS standards), 21
Nonverbal communication, 45–46
Nunch'i, 46

O

Oral Health in America, 20

P

Patients
  ethnocentrism in, 39, 40
  family as, 56
  indirect communication from, 47
  and linear time, 50, 52
  study on, 55–58
Payer, Lynn, 58–60, 73
Physicians, study on, 55–58
Polychronic(holistic) time orientation, 48, 77
Prescriptions. *See* Medications, prescriptions

R

Rao, Nagesh, 55–57, 73
Refugees, 55n27, 66–72, 77
Resources, 79

S

Smile, meaning of, 72
Soul loss, 68, 69
Southeast Asia, healthcare in, 66–72
Sumner, William, 38, 40
Supernatural illness, 68

T

Terrain, 62, 77
Thiederman, Sondra, 34
Time, cultural, 49–53
Transforming the Face of Health Professions Through Cultural and Linguistic Competence Education, 21

U

United States, healthcare in, 60–61, 66

V

Vandello, J., 44
Verbal communication, 45–48
Vietnamese, 69, 71–72

W

Wastebasket diagnosis
   constipation as, 65
   defined, 59–60, 77
   heart problems as, 63
   liver crisis as, 62
   virus as, 61
When "Yes" Means "No," 66
Wolfe, Thomas, 29

About the Author

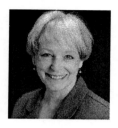

Toni Adams, who enjoys writing and giving presentations about communication topics for dental audiences, has won awards for writing, speaking, mentoring, scholarship, and leadership.

Toni practiced dental hygiene in and around San Jose, California, for 26 years. After "retirement," she earned baccalaureate and master's degrees in Communication Studies. She is interested in a broad range of communication topics including health, intercultural, and instructional communication, listening, persuasion, patient education, interviewing, and working with low literate and limited English proficient patients and interpreters.

She has taught college-level public speaking courses, has presented papers at communication conventions, has written articles for a variety of dental publications, is a member of Phi Kappa Phi national academic honor society, has worked as a Subject Matter Expert to help develop the California Dental Hygiene Law and Ethics examination, has served on several Editorial Advisory Boards, and was selected the 2009 Sonicare *RDH Magazine* Mentor of the Year.

Toni is also a wife of 42 years, mother of two fine sons, and grandmother of a brilliant and beautiful 6-year-old granddaughter.

Order Form

PLEASE PRINT CLEARLY

Book Selection	Quantity	Total @ $16 each
Book 1: Health Communication and Persuasion in Dentistry		
Book 2: Intercultural Communication in Dentistry		
Book 3: Verbal Communication in Dentistry		
Book 4: Nonverbal Communication in Dentistry		
Book 5: Listening in Dentistry		
Book 6: Patient Interviewing in Dentistry		
Book 7: Patient Education in Dentistry		
Totals (price includes tax)		$
Add Shipping & Handling (see chart on reverse)		$
Total enclosed (check or money order) Payable to: Odontocomm Productions Mail to: Odontocomm, P. O. Box 981, Rocklin, CA 95677		$

Complete shipping information on the other side of this form.

2-1

PLEASE PRINT CLEARLY

Mail books to (no Post Office Boxes, please):

Name: _____

Number/Street/Apt.# _____

_____

City/State/ZIP _____

_____

And, in case we need to contact you:

Phone with area code _____

Email address _____

_____

Shipping & Handling Costs

1 book	$5.00	8-14 books	$18.00
2-4 books	$9.00	15 or more books	FREE
5-7 books	$14.00		

Allow 4-6 weeks for delivery.

Do you have questions about:
Specials for students & instructors?
Large orders? Rush orders? Anything else?

Contact Toni for prices and shipping/handling costs.
office: 916.632.9848; cell: 916.316.5161
email: tonisadamsrdh@earthlink.net

Thank you for your order!

Order Form

PLEASE PRINT CLEARLY

Book Selection	Quantity	Total @ $16 each
Book 1: Health Communication and Persuasion in Dentistry		
Book 2: Intercultural Communication in Dentistry		
Book 3: Verbal Communication in Dentistry		
Book 4: Nonverbal Communication in Dentistry		
Book 5: Listening in Dentistry		
Book 6: Patient Interviewing in Dentistry		
Book 7: Patient Education in Dentistry		
Totals (price includes tax)		$
Add Shipping & Handling (see chart on reverse)		$
Total enclosed (check or money order) Payable to: Odontocomm Productions Mail to: Odontocomm, P. O. Box 981, Rocklin, CA 95677		$

Complete shipping information on the other side of this form.

2-1

PLEASE PRINT CLEARLY

Mail books to (no Post Office Boxes, please):

Name: _____

Number/Street/Apt.# _____

_____

City/State/ZIP _____

_____

And, in case we need to contact you:

Phone with area code _____

Email address _____

_____

Shipping & Handling Costs

1 book	$5.00	8-14 books	$18.00
2-4 books	$9.00	15 or more books	FREE
5-7 books	$14.00		

Allow 4-6 weeks for delivery.

**Do you have questions about:
Specials for students & instructors?
Large orders? Rush orders? Anything else?**

Contact Toni for prices and shipping/handling costs.
office: 916.632.9848; cell: 916.316.5161
email: tonisadamsrdh@earthlink.net

Thank you for your order!